How to Be Healthy & Have More Energy

A Guide to Optimum Wellness

By: Kevin Kerr

You should consult your physician or other health care professional before making any lifestyle or nutritional changes that are discussed, in order to determine if the suggested practices are right for your needs.

©2014, Kevin Kerr

All Rights Reserved.

Table of Contents

Introduction

With today's knowledge and understanding I believe we should all be living well past ninety years of age or more, especially considering the oldest living woman is now a hundred and twenty seven years old! If your desire is to feel and look your best then the willingness to make changes in your everyday routines must be present first. You are the creator of your reality. If you're not happy with your life it's because you are letting your mind tell you that you are not happy. Your thoughts control your actions which in turn create the way you look and feel. If you want to alter your lifestyle for your benefit or accomplish something new it can only be done if you learn to let go of doubtful thoughts. You can have anything and everything your heart desires!

This book is designed to start by helping you change your mindset which will in turn guide you toward optimal wellness. If you want to heal your body from the inside out from anything that you are suffering with whether it be physical, emotional, or spiritual, including all the toxins that we have been accumulating from birth, then I am here to help you accomplish your wishes. As simple as it may sound you have the power to heal your mind, body, and spirit if you just believe! The roots of all physical disease stem from the thoughts you think, toxicity and nutrient deficiencies. Three issues that can be alleviated very easily once the proper awareness is gained.

If you want to lose weight for good or gain weight then I can teach you how to do so if you are truly willing to make the necessary adjustments from within. Depending on how bad you truly want these changes correlates directly to how fast you will see real results. So basically what I mean is that you must believe in yourself as well as envision what you want to be, and practice feeling how you want to feel. It is important to start by consistently but slowly implementing the modifications discussed so they become habits, and every day you will feel better and have more and more energy as time goes on. Participating in simply half of these lifestyle techniques will add many years to your life along with those around you. I'm writing this because I care about you, and everyone else on this planet.

Meditation and Mindset

Before anything, the first step is to believe in yourself as well as be confident that you can achieve and deserve to have radiant health. You must believe that you can have unlimited energy, because after all you come from it and are made of it. Although the oldest woman on the planet attributes her longevity to her consumption of chocolate, which is considerably valid due to the fact that raw cacao (the plant source from which chocolate is made of) has more antioxidants than any other food; becoming aware of your breathing is probably the next best concept to master due to the fact that it takes your mind away from taxing thoughts which drain you of energy as well as supplies your cells with oxygen which is the most abundant mineral on earth. As odd as this may sound studies have shown that the fewer calories you consume the longer you live.

Whether we are aware of it most of us have dominate thought patterns and habits, which can make it hard for us to break self-destructive routines. Underneath all the chattering of the mind lies silence, once you let go of all thoughts, that will allow you to feel true bliss and peace of mind. If you continue to let your ego run your existence rather than feeling your way through each day then you will continue to get the same results in all areas of your life as well as feel the way you always do.

The first task to optimum wellness is to identify all the matters that are holding you back and write them down, and then come up with a list that will cure you from these ailments. Don't focus on the list that you have trouble with because if you do you will only get more of that. Keep the list of the tasks that you want more of. For example, if you watch too much TV then maybe you might want to walk more. Another issue could be your weight. If you want to lose weight it might not be that you eat too much, but not enough of the right types of food. The right balance of whole foods will get you where you want to be. Write down whatever it is you want to achieve or become. Don't let doubt come into your life. Be all that you want to be and always believe in yourself.

Meditation is something that you can practice everywhere all the time. You can be in a play of peace while still going about your day to day activities. You can allow God to run your life while you sit back and enjoy the show. You are infiniteness. You are God. If you make time to sit and be with your thoughts you will eventually have complete control over them which will help you in all areas of your life. If you start a meditation practice don't set a time frame, as it is just a man-made illusion, but try to do it consistently on a daily basis to ensure ensuring beneficial results.

The ego typically tries or wants to control everything in its path, but you have the power to let go of it. You have control over everything that you do as well as your reactions to everything that happens throughout your stay on this earth. Our ego labels events, material items as situations as good or bad pertaining to what it wants or does not want.

One way to get into a deep meditation is when you eat your food. A lot of people hardly chew their food several times before they swallow it which doesn't allow them to breakdown all the carbohydrates, fats, proteins, vitamins and minerals which causes them to be overweight, malnourished, or results in acne. This used to be a very big problem of mine. Train your brain to think "chew your food" while you eat. The more you chew your food the less you will eat and the more energy you will manifest. Eventually you can get so good at it that you will go into a state of meditation. If you drink smoothies or fresh fruit or vegetable juices then it's beneficial to swish it in your mouth to mix it with your saliva before you swallow to help initiate digestion before it reaches the stomach.

Lastly, I want to talk about sexual energy and I can't emphasize the importance of this enough when it comes to well-being. Master your sexual energy! We are receivers and transmitters of unseen forces. Life is infinite in a physical and metaphysical aspect. Say you give someone a compliment; this in turn sends them some positive energy that they in turn keep sharing to others throughout the day. This is relevant to sexual energy in that if you focus on it you can shift this energy to other areas of your life that need attention. Try going months without exerting this life-force. Focus on true unconditional love which is the love of all of God's creations. A clear picture and a burning desire of what you want must be instilled within your mind so that everyday distractions do not get in the way of its accomplishment. We are meant to create even if it doesn't happen every time we have sex, and it takes a lot of energy to create another living being. If we take our focus off the usual intentional failed attempts at creation we can redirect our energy towards the things we want, and actually manifest them as quick as you imagine them. The following is a list of strategies and tips that will help you achieve the proper mindset for achieving optimal health as well as more energy:

- you are the creator of your reality
- you have the power to change your thoughts
- your thoughts determine the way you look and feel
- let go of doubtful thoughts
- stay in the moment as much as

possible
- become conscious of your breathing
- look at life through your peripherals

Hydration

A lot of people would agree that they need to drink more water on a daily basis. There really is no particular way to do anything in life, but there is always room for improvement. I weigh around a hundred and fifty pounds and I generally drink at least a gallon of water a day which is a hundred and twenty eight ounces or sixteen cups. Some experts recommend drinking an ounce per pound of bodyweight per day. I can almost guarantee that if you slowly incorporate more into your diet you will continually have more energy day after day.

So many individuals are dehydrated, and don't know what it feels like to be hydrated because they never have been. The lack of water causes the inside of their bodies to be sticky because of the deficiency of water in the cells. Slowly work your way up to drinking more until you find what works best for you, but don't force anything. Organic coconut water is a great way to speed up the process because they are high in electrolytes which allow your cells to take in the water. If you have access to young green coconuts this can be a great way to take your health and hydration to a new level.

Clean water is what your body craves. I think that many people don't drink enough water because they don't have access to clean water and aren't even aware of it. Chemically treated tap water from your city is some of the most toxic water on the planet. Any filter is better than no filter, or you can gather your water from a reliable spring which can be found at findaspring.com. True spring water is so valuable because it comes from very deep depths, making it very clean and bioavailable for the cells. I prefer spring water but if I don't have access to it I opt for the best water I can find. The three best filters next to Mother Nature are a reverse osmosis system, a water distiller, or a gravity filter. Drink only when you are thirsty. Do what makes you feel best. You may look back one day and realize it was one of the best decisions you've ever made like I have.

There are several ways that you can jumpstart the hydration process which I highly recommend. The first is always drink water before you eat meals, and especially when you wake up. This will also aid in digestion. Without the proper amount of potassium and sodium in your body your body's cells won't be able to intake the extra water you are putting in your system. All raw foods are high in potassium, the common one probably being bananas. Most people get plenty of salt in their diet but it is important to find your balance of potassium and sodium for proper hydration.

Squeezing a half of or a whole lemon into a cup of water when you rise first thing in the morning is another valuable method for achieving optimal wellness and hydration. Every day I consume one lemon and one avocado. Lemon water triggers the liver to secrete bile which helps break down food, resulting in fabulous digestion. Studies have shown that if you use warm water it is more effective. I store all my water on the counter rather than the fridge because it takes unnecessary energy to heat cold water up to your body's temperature. If you can't drink lemon water because it is too bitter then I suggest drinking it with stevia powder or liquid extract. It's an herb that has no negative effects on the human body, making it the safest sweetener known to man. If you desire sugar then opt for organic due to the fact that conventional is made from genetically modified beets, making them very toxic to the human body. Coconut sugar or lo han guo are other safer alternatives as well.

The last, but most effective, cellular hydration technique I want to share with you is juicing. Smoothies are great, and I'll admit that I do consume most of the water I drink in smoothies, but juices are a whole level of health. Consuming fresh homemade fruit and vegetable juices provides your body with truly bioavailable nutrition due to the fact that there is no fiber to break down. If you've never had a juice then I suggest starting with carrots and celery which are high in potassium and sodium. Greens vegetables are some of the most nutrient dense foods to juice, and they mix well with apples to take away the bitterness. Juicing is so beneficial for the body because it is full of micronutrients. Many people are getting plenty of macronutrients which include carbohydrates, fats, and proteins. Micronutrients are all the minerals that your body needs to run optimally. There are around ninety different minerals that the human body needs many of which in incredibly small amounts. However, the conventional food supply only puts three different minerals back into the soil. This causes the body to become unbalanced. If you don't have a juicer you can invest in a cheap one for less than thirty dollars. I got my first two that were used for less than five dollars apiece. Best investments of my life!

Exercise and Grounding

A little bit of exercise goes a long way. You don't need to overwork your body at the gym to be in peak physical condition. Simply moving more and walking can be the best exercise protocol. Exercising is one of the most effective ways to boost your metabolism, burn unwanted belly fat, and remove toxins from the body.

I have found that taking regular walks on daily basis keeps my body in peak physical condition. Walking in the morning before you eat breakfast is a great start to getting healthier and detoxifying your body because right when you wake up your body is in the peak stage of detoxification. So if you wait an hour or two before eating you will extend and intensify the detox and fat burning mechanisms of your body.

Grounding and inverting are two exercises that are immensely life prolonging for the human body and incredibly simple as well as free. Ground is simply getting barefoot contact with the earth to recharge all the cells and inverting is putting the human body upside down to alleviate the effects of gravity. If you are not capable of headstands or handstands then you can lean your body over the armrest of a couch. Doing this for ten minutes counterbalances a whole day's worth of the harmful effects of gravity. It also stimulates the lymphatic system which is waste removal pathway of the body. It brings more blood to the brain and makes you feel great!

Grounding or earthing is a wonderful way to revitalize the entire system. There is a book entitled *Earthing* that I highly recommended which explains the scientific details of this practice. It has helped numerous individuals heal from all sorts of health ailments. It alleviates the effects of electromagnetic frequencies from today's technology and allows the cells to communicate to aid in detoxification and repair. If you want to invest some money in your health you can purchase a grounding device for when you sleep and/or an inversion table to help with inverting.

Aside from taking long walks, my favorite exercise is breathing. The best time to practice this is during times of meditation, while you are waiting for something or someone, or all day if you can manage it. Being aware of your breathing takes you from your thoughts and supplies your body with the with more energy than food or drink. Diaphragmatic breathing allows you to get more oxygen for less breath. The way to go about this is to breathe in through your nose into your stomach. If you take a big enough breath you can make your belly protrude. Next, breathe this air into your lungs, and then exhale. This method of breathing can make a huge difference in your health.

Non-Toxic Lifestyle

Don't expect to become enlightened in the dark of the night. The sun provides us with food and our bodies with energy. Exposure to it works synergistically with the skin to produce vitamin D, which is actually classified as a hormone. Hormones create our behaviors and moods. The benefits of sun exposure are being more documented as the days go on but it has been known to cure depression and eliminate harmful bacteria from the body. Aim for at least thirty minutes a day but you should spend as much time in the sun as you are able to. Increasing your exposure can greatly improve your overall well-being and longevity.

If you haven't already come to the realization that nearly every conventional product is toxic and disrupting to the body's hormone producing systems, then I'm here to help you become aware of this. There are natural products that you can buy or make at home as I do. I love you use Google to find homemade non-toxic recipes. Making your own is not only cheaper, but way healthier! Baking soda, coconut oil, essential oils for scent, shea butter, vinegars, along with vodka all work wonders in whatever combination your heart desires for deodorants, dish soap, laundry detergent, toothpaste, and any self or home cleansing remedies you might need. Lastly, if you live in a city then I want to recommend a shower de-chlorinator. Chlorine is great for the treatment of pathogens but it is toxic to the human. When it reacts with hot water in your shower it creates a gas that is breathed in. You can purchase a high quality one for less than fifty dollars at freedrinkingwater.com.

Sometimes it's necessary to let go of toxic relationships. If you feel as if the people you hang out with are holding you back from evolving spiritually then it's okay to move on because you can always keep them in your heart; if it's what you need then might be beneficial for them as well. Everything that happens in life is necessary for the evolution of consciousness. It may be hard to see sometimes but it is all love.

A good relationship is one that is constantly giving and receiving acts of love. One that is working to rid the body of toxins rather than accumulating them. Although you are responsible for your own inner-circumstance and decisions, until you become fully present it is often easy to become like the people you hang out with. If you are in a close relationship with someone who is self-destructive, and you aware of this then love yourself and move on if you feel as if they are bringing you down.

What to Eat and When

For some reason I've noticed that people struggle most when it comes to eating healthy. I suppose we could attribute it to the abundance of genetically engineered, fast, and processed food in grocery stores. The best way to overcome this is to simply throw out all the food that you know is harmful in your house and replace it with foods made of love. The first step is become aware as to what is optimal for the human body. However, at the end of the day something is only going to harm you if you think it is, but when you make a conscious decision to eat healthy organic food it will be abundantly inexpensive for everyone. This will in turn make the world a better place for all of us.

If you want to see fast weight loss results and better health then try switching to a ketogenic diet or in other words an intermittent fasting regime. People who partake in this discipline have amazing results. The method to this diet is to eat within a specific time frame, generally around eight hours out of the day or less. It retrains your body to use fat as an energy source rather than carbs. Another way to improve your health is to stop eating before six or seven p.m. every night to allow optimal digestion and nutrient assimilation.

Science is quickly proving that a plant-based diet is more optimal for the human body. I choose to eat an all raw vegan diet because I've done the research and it can be the healthiest lifestyle if done properly. I find it most optimal for my body. If you desire radiant health then I recommend learning everything you need to know about it before transitioning to this diet. I've read that if humans all became herbivores there would be enough food to feed the entire planet sevenfold, curing starvation. In order for your body to break down food to convert it into energy it must produce digestive enzymes. It takes eighty percent of the bodies energy do this, and the studies show that your body can only produce so many digestive enzymes within one lifespan. Raw plant foods contain digestive enzymes. The fresher they are the more enzymes they contain. If you want quick long lasting energy that will give you energy all day, without the crash, then reach for the fruit and/or raw foods. If you want to lose weight, no matter how much you eat, and have more energy than you've ever had then try transitioning to a raw plant-based diet. It is also very possible to gain weight on a raw vegan diet if you increase your fat and protein intake with intense training and/or weight lifting. They have done studies on the longest-lived people and what they like to eat. The top five longevity foods as a collective include all vegetarian sources as followed: chocolate, cinnamon, red onions, olive oil, and honey. Whatever you eat, opt for organic or homegrown and preferably raw.

Organic foods are important for a number of reasons. They cannot be irradiated or produced with toxic chemicals such as pesticides, herbicides, fungicides, or larvicides. They also cannot be grown from genetically modified seeds. Irradiation is a food preservation process that destroys all the healthy bacteria which is important for the human body; it also has been proven to destroy vital nutrients. Local and homegrown organic fresh fruits and vegetables are the safest as well as most nutritious food options. I eat an avocado a day to help curve nutrient deficiencies because it is such a complete food source. If you've never had one, or don't like them try one with cold pressed olive oil and sea or pink Himalayan salt. It is my favorite food combination. Herbs are so beneficial for the human body. Taking herbs on a daily basis ensure optimum health and help to curb viruses, fungus, and bacteria that are trying to take over the human body. There are thousands to choose from! I love herbs! To end the book, I am going to leave you with a list of foods, minerals, and products of nature that will help you with the detox and remineralization process:

- Organic Whole Foods
- Activated Coconut Charcoal
- Aloe Vera
- Avocados
- Bee Pollen
- Bentonite Clay
- Berries (Organic and/or Wild)
- B-Vitamin Complex (Especially sublingual b 12)
- Chia Seeds
- Coffee (Organic and preferably shade grown)
- Chlorella
- Digestive Enzymes
- Essential Fatty Acids
- Fulvic Acid
- Green Vegetables and Herbs (The more the merrier)
- Hemp Seeds
- Iodine
- Maca
- Magnesium
- Marine Phytoplankton
- Medicinal Mushrooms (Specifically Chaga and Reishi)
- MSM
- Olive Oil (Cold pressed)
- Probiotics and/or Fermented Foods
- Raw Cacao (Chocolate)
- Sea Vegetables
- Shilajit
- Spirulina

- Wild Foods
- Zeolite Clay

www.ingramcontent.com/pod-product-compliance
Lightning Source LLC
Chambersburg PA
CBHW071349310526
45790CB00018B/1395